YOUR KNOWLEDGE HAS VALUE

Charles Ross

Stroke service. Helping in emergencies

GRIN Verlag

Bibliografische Information der Deutschen Nationalbibliothek:

Die Deutsche Bibliothek verzeichnet diese Publikation in der Deutschen National-
bibliografie; detaillierte bibliografische Daten sind im Internet über http://dnb.d-
nb.de/ abrufbar.

Imprint:

Copyright © 2010 GRIN Verlag GmbH
Druck und Bindung: Books on Demand GmbH, Norderstedt Germany
ISBN: 978-3-656-61096-0

This book at GRIN:

http://www.grin.com/en/e-book/269786/stroke-service-helping-in-emergencies

GRIN - Your knowledge has value

Der GRIN Verlag publiziert seit 1998 wissenschaftliche Arbeiten von Studenten, Hochschullehrern und anderen Akademikern als eBook und gedrucktes Buch. Die Verlagswebsite www.grin.com ist die ideale Plattform zur Veröffentlichung von Hausarbeiten, Abschlussarbeiten, wissenschaftlichen Aufsätzen, Dissertationen und Fachbüchern.

Visit us on the internet:

http://www.grin.com/

http://www.facebook.com/grincom

http://www.twitter.com/grin_com

Stroke Service - Helping in emergencies

Overview

For those who are having issues with their heart and have serious heart ailments can always avail the stroke services which are equipped with all the necessary aspects that will help you in saving your life. The service of stroke team is considered the best and is available in different parts of this globe. Along with providing diagnosis, treatment and prevention, proper care is provided to the patients who are having cerebrovascular ailments. As strokes are considered one of the most hazardous ailments to take life of a person, both private and public sector hospitals are offering the services of stroke teams so that they can eradicate the fear of stroke for a person when they are alone at their home without any assistance. Over the years, medical industry has seen several changes and has brought out the best of what medical wonder can do. Working in the medical industry is a dream for every individual as it is not just a best paying job, but it even gives an urge to serve the people who are in need.

Strokes Services- Better working possibilities in the private sector

Stokes services have become popular in different ways as it is only dedicated to those who are having heart ailments. The stroke services can be availed at home and even at the hospital centers as in British Stroke Association. When a person is having a symptom of stroke, they are transported to an emergency department after which the strokes service is provided to them. The people who are associated in the strokes service team have always stated that they are proud to be in such a team because they are able to help the person in need. (Andersen et. al, 2002)

The need of emergency stroke services has increased, it has become one of the hottest job sectors, which is selected by professionals who are working or want to be a part of the medical industry. It does not matter if the hospital in which you are working is a private or public center, because the result is always the service that you are providing. The strokes services have been divided into different parts so that it is easy to handle a case in a best possible manner. Along with this, as varieties of professionals are there, they are able to work accordingly by playing their part to help a person having a stroke. The diagnosis is being done and the treatment follows suit in a rapid force when the strokes service team takes the thing in their hands. (Healthcare Commission, 2006)

Availing strokes services at home as a precaution

At times, it happens that the near and dear ones are diagnosed with some terminal heart illness. This is the most crucial time for the family, as they have to decide whether they have to keep their beloved with themselves or not. It is very tough to leave your most loved people at hospitals and nursing homes especially at times when they are ill and need your presence. However, it is not possible to stay with them all the time and this puts you in dilemma of what to do. If you are one among those who wish to see your loved ones in front of your eyes and wish to take part in their treatment strokes services is just the perfect solution to all your problems.

Guidelines that has to be followed- The key national policies and guidelines relevant to the delivery of this service

Numerous institutes and companies that provide short time registered courses provide strokes services to the people. You can visit any such organization and hire one for your family. British Stroke Association is the one organization where most of the strokes service specialists have training and certification of registered nursing course and they have knowledge about providing ailments and dealing with people suffering from heart illness. You can get their detailing and qualification from the hospitals. However, there are certain rules and laws that are made by the government to maintain a healthy relationship between both the parties. For this, you should seek a lawyer and get an agreement signed on paper. This agreement generally deals with the perquisites and facilities that you will be providing to the strokes service personal as well as the areas of duty and responsibility that they will be fulfilling. The method of payment as well as the term for which the person is employed is also mentioned in the agreement. A copy of it is also submitted at the nearby police station for complete security and assurance. (Geddes & Chamberlain, 2001)

Many advantages accompany the hiring of strokes services at home. This might include factors like fast recovery due to homely environment. The best thing about them is that you can see you loved ones in front of yourself and can participate in their treatment. This is the most sought advantage as one might be spending hours in travelling to hospitals and nursing homes everyday to see their loved ones. This might also leave them unaware of the everyday progress of the patient as well as the current health conditions.

The role of key personnel who are involved in delivering this service

Having a strokes service at home provides assurance on medical as well as on emotional grounds as one is satisfied with the fact that their loved one is getting the best service and treatment and shall be well in some time. If you are having your loved one suffering from any kind of chronic, terminal or any other type of disease related to heart you can choose this service for them. It is not very costly as well and saves the extra money that you might be spending at getting treatments from hospital. Whether the person suffering from heart ailments is a child or an adult these practitioners from the strokes service provide equally well assistance to both.

4

For a person who is availing the strokes services have to follow some particular guidelines that would are designed for the betterment of their health. Once a case is handled by the strokes service team, they have to look into the case and do the necessary arrangements of all the tests that are to be conducted so that a proper diagnosis can be done for treatment. The stroke specialist is looking after all the things related to the strokes service. Reason behind this is that, they are having the experience and knowledge in handling the cases in the best possible manner. The key personals looking after the strokes services are mostly neurosurgeons who know how to handle the critical issues with care. In addition to this, there are even cardio experts and surgeons who can look after the heart stroke cases.

The role of regulatory bodies on the quality of the service provided and the impact of non-conformity

Even the hospitals, which are offering the strokes services have some rules and regulations, that has to be followed by all the professionals. With help of these rules and regulations, the stroke service professionals are able to give their best in performing their duties in the desired manner. In addition to this, there are certain regulatory bodies, which are managing the strokes services in the best possible manner. The regulatory bodies for the strokes services have clearly made a point that they want to give the best services to people who are having any form of heart ailment. The chief medical officer of the private medical institutes is looking after all the working of the strokes services along with which makes the amendments accordingly.

The current political agenda, available funding and influence the service. (Funds and political agendas of the strokes services)

Mostly all the funds are allocated by the governing authorities of the hospitals. As strokes services is an important part of the hospitals, they ate spending a hefty amount for the betterment of the strokes services. Along with this, new reforms and changes are always done on a constant basis depending on the political agendas of the hospitals. With the political agendas changing from time to time, they are even offering changes for funds so that it suits the requirement of the strokes services and even the hospitals. (Fahey et. al, 2003)

The impact on strokes services-The society point of view

As strokes services are getting handy for the users, the people are opting for the same on the large. According to different research programs and analysis, it was found that people in the society are now open to the strokes services as an awareness regarding the same is being created. For a person who is having heart ailments, the strokes services has come like a boon as they are diagnosed in a proper manner after which the process of treatment is started. In addition to this, as the whole work is done in an organized manner and by the specialists, the faith over the strokes services has increased with time.

The trust and believe of the society over the services has even given a boost to the strokes services to work on a positive note and safe lives. With this motivation and availability of funds from the hospitals, the strokes service is being enhanced into new ways so that quality of the service is maintained. Another point that makes strokes service popular amidst the society is the help that they provide for a person to recover from the shock of having a stroke. Depending on the needs, some rehabilitation service is even provided along with the strokes services.

The impact of new technology on the service provided

As time is running on the fast lane, technological changes are done at a rapid pace. With the changes in technology, the strokes services have been enhanced in a new way. Today, the hospitals, which are offering the strokes services at home, can do the diagnosis and tests in a hassle free manner. In addition to this, even the ambulances are now being equipped with special equipments and other necessary tools that will help the patient who is having a stroke.

With the changes coming on at a rapid pace, the professionals who are associated with the strokes services are learning new concepts and methods that can make the working easy and simple. Even the health facility centers are having the best and the finest equipments so that they can give the best strokes services to the patients 24*7. With the changes in technology, the strokes service team can judge and detect the problem within a snap of time. With advanced forms of technology, the strokes service team would now be able to detect the actual place of the stroke so that similar proceedings can be conducted to help the patient.

As technological development has gone to new levels, the people associated with offering the strokes service are now having the tools and equipments that can detect the symptoms of having a stroke; this will help in preventing the same. Vascular malformations along with aneurysms are the two main forms of strokes that can now be avoided and controlled with the technological changes that have come into existence. Below mentioned are some of the advanced equipments that are used while providing strokes services.

Neurovascular ultrasound: This test is conducted with high frequencies of sound waves to detect the issues with the artillery walls, which can create a stroke.

Magnetic Resonance image (MRI): With use of this technological wonder, exact images of the internal organs are being designed which even shows the tissues that ate damages and can cause a stroke.

MRA: With use of this technology, the blood vessels in the body are calculated and proper treatment is being advised if they are found to be low.

SPECT: Single photon emission computerized tomographs are being used to generate 3D images of the brain and heart so that main reasons of the stroke are being known. This is one of the most advanced tools being used while providing the strokes services.

Along with this, if a person is given strokes services are home, then EKG, EEG and ECG along with EPS is easily possible because now the equipments for doing these tests have become portable and handy. (Elkind, 2005)

Conclusion

The strokes service has become one of the most used methods by the hospitals for specially looking after the people who are suffering from any ailment that can cause a stroke. In addition to this, it has proved to be a great impact on the society as people have attained success from the stroke services. Considering this, the political agendas have changed and the governing bodies who are involved in making the rules and regulations have sanctioned big amounts so that best facilities can be provided. Last but not the least, the advancement of technology has helped strokes services in a great way. Today, modernized machines and tools are available that can be used while offering strokes service to save a life of a person.

References:

Andersen HE, Eriksen K, Brown A, Schutz-Larsen K, Forchammer BH. (2002). Follow-up services for stroke survivors after hospital discharge - a randomised control trial. Clinical Rehabilitation; 16: 593-603

Elkind MS. (2005). Implications of stroke prevention trials: treatment of global risk. Neurology; 65 (1):

Fahey T, Montgomery AA, Barnes J, Protheroe J. (2003). Quality of care for elderly residents in nursing homes and elderly people living at home: controlled observational study. British Medical Journal; 326: 580.

Geddes JML, Chamberlain MA. (2001). Home-based rehabilitation for people with stroke: a comparative study of six community services providing coordinated multidisciplinary treatment. Clinical Rehabilitation; 15: 589-599.

Healthcare Commission. (2006) Caring for people after they have had a stroke. A follow-up survey of patients. http://www.healthcarecommission.org.uk/_db/_documents/stroke_survey_update.pdfAccessed February 11th 2008